CAREERS IN

RHEUMATOLOGY

DOCTORS TREATING ARTHRITIS AND AUTOIMMUNE DISEASES AFFECTING MILLIONS OF PEOPLE

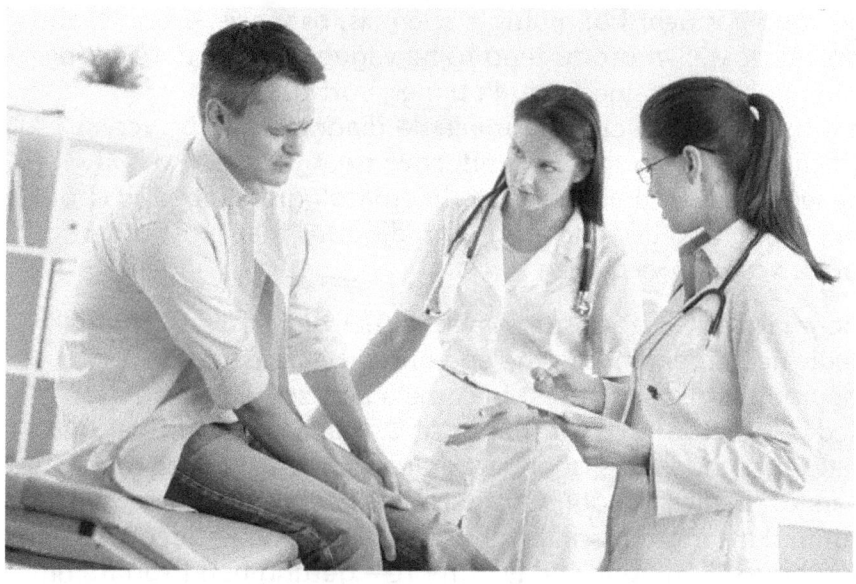

RHEUMATOLOGY IS THE BRANCH OF MEDICINE dealing with musculoskeletal disorders and autoimmune diseases. There are more than 200 of these rheumatic diseases, afflicting millions of Americans of all ages. By far, the most common disease treated by rheumatologists is arthritis. According to the CDC (Center For

Disease Control), arthritis alone affects more than 53 million people, or 23 percent of all adults in the US!

Osteoarthritis is the leading form of arthritis, but there are others, such as rheumatoid arthritis, gout, and lupus. In fact, there are 100 different kinds of arthritis. They all cause pain, aching, stiffness, and swelling in or around the joints. Some can affect multiple organs and create life threatening conditions. Some may be acute, while others are chronic, meaning they last a lifetime.

Rheumatology is also concerned with autoimmune diseases that afflict roughly 50 million Americans. There are many kinds of autoimmune diseases. Most have unfamiliar names, but nearly everyone has heard of multiple sclerosis, psoriasis, Crohn's, and fibromyalgia. Symptoms tend to be vague, such as unrelenting fatigue or unexplained pain in bones, soft tissue, or gastrointestinal tract. Determining a diagnosis can be very difficult. Choosing the most effective treatment is also challenging. But that is what a rheumatologist's job is all about – diagnosing and treating long-term diseases that most other doctors cannot recognize.

Rheumatology is a subspecialty of either pediatrics or internal medicine, depending on the age group being treated. Rheumatologists must first become a licensed physician – Medical Doctor (MDs) or Doctor of Osteopathic Medicine (DO). That takes four years of undergraduate college followed by four years of medical school. Another three years of residency is required after graduating from medical school. Residents put in long hours – 16 hours a day or more – getting hands-on training in a hospital setting. After that, their skills are perfected in fellowship programs that typically last an additional two to four years. Rheumatologists who start their educational path right after high school are well into their thirties by the time they are qualified to start practicing on their own.

With such a heavy investment in education, it is good to know that it is going to be worth it. Rheumatologists report a high degree of satisfaction in their careers. In fact, rheumatologists are known as the happiest specialists. The work is intellectually stimulating, highly rewarding, and the earnings are excellent averaging well over $200,000 a year.

The job outlook is excellent, too. Nationwide, there are more openings than candidates to fill them, and that gap is widening. Most rheumatologists work in hospitals and clinics, but many are also employed by assisted care facilities, government health agencies, private health organizations, universities, and pharmaceutical companies. Those who are not employed as salaried staff are in private practice. They often see patients who have been referred by primary care physicians. Many are affiliated with hospitals, acting as consultants when hospitalized patients show signs of rheumatic disease.

Becoming a rheumatologist means being in a position to alleviate pain and enhance the quality of life for people. If you have a strong interest in physiology, have an aptitude for solving problems, possess excellent communications skills, and want to help people, take a closer look. Rheumatology may be the career you are looking for.

WHAT YOU CAN DO NOW

A CAREER IN RHEUMATOLOGY requires a rigorous education. Start preparing for college admission requirements early in high school. Take as many science and math classes as you can. The most important are biology, chemistry, physics, algebra, and calculus. Any other classes in natural sciences or health-related subjects are big pluses. Communications are extremely important in this career. Develop your reading, writing and speaking skills through English literature, speech, and debate classes. You will be working with people from all walks of life. Learning a foreign language and taking a psychology class will be very helpful.

To make sure rheumatology is a good fit for you, talk to professionals in the field. Contact your local hospital or rheumatology clinic and ask to talk to the rheumatologist. Most will be happy to give you an inside look at what their work entails. Arrange for a job shadow. A full day or two will provide an inside look at a typical day. Be prepared to ask a lot of questions about what to expect in school, and what they like and dislike about their work.

A part-time job in healthcare is an ideal way to determine if medicine is your calling. It does not have to be in rheumatology. Any position in healthcare will be helpful. If you cannot find a paying job, volunteer at the local hospital. In addition to providing valuable experience, it will look good on your college entrance application.

Spend some time on the Internet. There are numerous professional associations for rheumatologists that provide information of interest to students. The American College of Rheumatology (ACR), in particular, focuses on education related to the field. Get in the habit of reading medical journals, too. You will be doing that continually throughout your career.

There are also some internships open to high school juniors and seniors, such as those offered by the Arthritis Foundation. Internships for high school students are usually eight weeks long and are scheduled to fit into summer vacation time. Internships provide hands-on experience through basic laboratory research or clinical patient-oriented research.

HISTORY OF THE PROFESSION

THE ORIGIN OF RHEUMATOLOGY CAN BE TRACED BACK to a time before modern humans populated the earth. When scientists examined the bones of Neanderthal Man, they discovered spinal arthritis. That means the disease has existed for at least 50,000 years!

Instances of arthritis have been recorded throughout history. Many ancient skeletons show signs of osteoarthritis and gout (a disorder that causes arthritis). The disease has also been found in the remains of medieval Saxon soldiers and Egyptian mummies. In fact, even Ramses II, was afflicted. It was the Egyptians who first identified gout, known as podagra, in 2640 BC. Descriptions of arthritis was recorded in *Ebers Papyrus,* written circa 1500 BC. Evidence of arthritis can also be found in many famous paintings of the Medieval Era.

In ancient India, renowned Ayurvedic physician, Charaka, wrote about arthritis around 300 BC. His book on Indian medicine, *Charaka Samhita*, defines many variants of arthritis along with vivid descriptions of symptoms, including pain, joint swelling, and loss of function. Hippocrates also described arthritis, about 2400 years ago. The ancient Greek physician offered several observations, mostly focusing on gout, which he called "the unwalkable disease." He pointed out that it was related to an affluent lifestyle and labeled it "arthritis of the rich."

The term rheumatology is rooted in the word "rheuma," which means flowing. The word dates back to the 1st century AD. In the 2nd century AD, Greek physician Galen, coined the term "rheumatismus." In the 16th century, the term was changed to its final form by French physician, Guillaume de Baillou. In his book, *The Book on Rheumatism and Back Pain,* he introduced the term "rheumatism."

Ancient Therapies

Various therapies have been used to treat rheumatic ailments throughout history. Ancient Egyptians and Assyrians used willow extract to reduce the redness and pain of inflamed joints. Hippocrates endorsed the use of laxatives and diet therapy, while Galen advocated barley water and barley bread. However, diet therapy was unsuccessful until about 10 AD, when Antonius Musa treated Roman Emperor Augustus with cold baths for a case of arthritis so severe, it crippled his hands and feet. Other therapies tried in ancient times included spa therapy (both cold and hot water), bloodletting, and counter irritants, such as Capsaicin, menthol, and camphor.

The use of anti-inflammatory agents, such as willow bark and salicin (a partially purified extract of willow bark), emerged in the 16th century. The active component of willow bark is salicylic acid, commonly known today as aspirin. Hammond Kolbe first synthesized salicylic acid in 1859. Aspirin has been used extensively ever since for the treatment of arthritis and rheumatic fever.

Rheumatology – a 20th Century Profession

Several important discoveries were made in 1948, mostly involving methods of diagnosis. The most successful was the development of a serological test for rheumatoid arthritis (RA). That same year, Philip Hench, a rheumatologist at Mayo Clinic, successfully treated an RA patient with a corticosteroid for the first time. The treatment was a major milestone in rheumatology. In 1950, Hench was awarded the Nobel Prize for Medicine for his discovery and its application for the treatment of RA.

Other treatments, such as the antimalarial drug, quinacrine, and chloroquine were used to treat arthritis in the 1950s. Hydroxychloroquine is still widely used today for the treatment of many rheumatic diseases. However, the next milestone did not come until 1968 when methotrexate was introduced. Methotrexate, which is chemically similar to folic acid, was developed by Yellapragada Subbarao, an Indian scientist working in the US. It was originally used as a chemotherapy treatment for cancer, but in much lower doses significantly reduces inflammation and decreases joint damage. After proving its efficacy in the treatment of rheumatic diseases, the FDA approved it in 1988. Low-dose methotrexate has since become the go-to drug for the treatment of many rheumatic and autoimmune diseases.

Rheumatology developed as a well-recognized specialty of medicine in the mid-20th century. American physician, Bernard Comroe, coined the term rheumatologist in 1940. The word rheumatology first appeared in a textbook written by another American doctor, Joseph Lee Hollander, in 1949.

Allopurinol was a new drug to be used in the treatment of gout. Physicians George Hitchings and Gertrude Elion used allopurinol successfully in 1963. In 1988, they shared the Nobel Prize in Medicine for their work in developing allopurinol, azathioprine, and five other drugs.

The 1990s saw a landmark development in the treatment of rheumatic diseases with the introduction of disease-modifying agents. Researchers Sir Ravinder Maini and Marc Feldmann were pioneers in the study of autoimmune diseases and disease-modifying antirheumatic drugs (DMARDs). They discovered the disease mechanism that drives key processes like inflammation, immunity, and cell growth. Their work led to a series of successful clinical trials using the DMARD infliximab, to suppress the body's overactive immune and/or inflammatory systems. For the first time, DMARDs made it possible to alter the underlying disease rather than simply treating symptoms. The success of Maini and Feldmann led to major pharmaceutical companies racing to market. By 1998, etanercept (Enbrel) was approved for treatment in the US, and by 1999, infliximab (Remicade) was also approved. Several more DMARDs have since been developed. DMARDs have become the therapy of choice not only for RA, but also for numerous autoimmune diseases including Crohn's disease, ulcerative colitis, ankylosing spondylitis, psoriasis, vasculitis, and psoriatic arthritis.

The field of rheumatology is continually progressing. Advances in molecular biology have helped rheumatologists better understand the disease process. Progress in immunology, genetics, and imaging have led to greatly improved diagnostics as well as new therapeutic targets such as inflammatory mediators. Medical science has gone from patients to tissues to cells and now to genetic precursors.

Today, rheumatologists play a vital role in American medicine. Virtually every branch of internal medicine interacts with rheumatology. There are more than 100 diseases specifically classified as rheumatic, including many types of arthritis. These diseases afflict more than 46 million people in the US, many of whom experience extreme pain and reduced mobility. They depend on rheumatologists to provide relief so they can lead normal lives.

Rheumatologists are also responsible for diagnosing and treating autoimmune diseases, which account for the fastest growing area of illness in the US. It represents a global problem, but in this country there are now 50 million Americans suffering from autoimmune diseases. That is roughly 20 percent of the population or one in five people who are diagnosed with diseases like lupus, celiac disease, fibromyalgia, Chrone's, and Type 1 diabetes.

People have been suffering for many thousands of years, but today's rheumatologists can provide accurate diagnoses and highly targeted therapies with very minor side effects. The field of rheumatology will surely develop even further in the future through better science.

WHERE YOU WILL WORK

THERE ARE ABOUT 5,200 RHEUMATOLOGISTS working in the US. Almost all of them work with adults. Most work in outpatient clinics. They are typically affiliated with a hospital and are expected to care for hospitalized patients who show indications of a rheumatic disease. Because rheumatic disorders are most common among the elderly, nursing homes, long-term care facilities, and retirement communities also employ rheumatologists. Other employers include:

- Community health centers
- Home health agencies
- Government health agencies
- Pharmaceutical companies
- Inpatient facilities that provide rehabilitation and transitional care
- Universities

Those who work in academia typically conduct research in addition to their teaching duties. Others conducting research may work in laboratories operated by pharmaceutical firms or in government facilities.

It is very common for rheumatologists to work in private practice. Some may be salaried employees, but that is usually only the case for new professionals starting out. Experienced rheumatologists either own their own practice or become a partner in a group practice.

Most professionals in this field provide direct patient care, but some do consulting, administration, training, or supervising. It is also common for rheumatologists to be involved in community service.

The primary work environment of a rheumatologist is a medical office or clinic. These places are well-lit, temperature controlled, and medically sterile.

Most rheumatologists work full time. Workweeks and total hours on the job vary, depending on the employer. Rheumatologists typically see at least 10 patients a day. Patient visits are scheduled 30 minutes apart, but consultations can go longer. Even though the schedule may look like a normal 40-hour week, it will usually end up being more like 60 hours. Those working in private practice only work during the week, Monday through Friday. Those working for hospitals, however, may be scheduled for weekends or holidays. They may also be on call.

THE WORK YOU WILL DO

A RHEUMATOLOGIST IS A DOCTOR who specializes in the treatment of musculoskeletal disorders and systemic autoimmune conditions, collectively referred to as rheumatic diseases. There are more than 200 different rheumatic disorders that affect the joints, bones, muscles, and soft tissues. Many affect multiple organ systems that may cause patients to confront life-threatening complications.

The most common rheumatic disease treated by rheumatologists is arthritis. This disorder alone affects more than 46 million adults in the US and over a quarter million children. There are more than 100 types of arthritis, but it is generally divided into two main types: osteoarthritis and rheumatoid arthritis (commonly referred to as RA). There are 10 times as many people with osteoarthritis than RA.

Osteoarthritis, also known as degenerative arthritis or OA, involves the inflammation, breakdown, and the eventual loss of cartilage in joints. It was once thought that it was caused by the natural wearing down of joints over time, but doctors now view it as a disease of the joints that can affect people of any age. The cause may be genetics, excessive weight, or injury and overuse. It is common in athletes, for example, to repeatedly damage joints, tendons, and ligaments, until the cartilage eventually breaks down. Osteoarthritis typically affects weight-bearing joints, such as the hips, knees, and spine. It can also affect non-weight bearing joints like the fingers, thumb, neck, and large toe. Osteoarthritis causes inflammation and pain in the affected joint, which is usually treated with anti-inflammatories.

Rheumatoid arthritis involves an abnormal inflammatory response, which makes it an autoimmune disorder. It often features stiffness and swelling in multiple joints accompanied by systemic symptoms, including fever, pain, or fatigue. While osteoarthritis typically affects only certain joints, RA is more systemic. It can cause a painful swelling in all or most joints at once. Symptoms tend to decrease as joints are used throughout the day. That is the opposite of osteoarthritis, where symptoms increase the more joints are used. Both RA and OA are treated with anti-inflammatory medications (NSAIDs), but RA may be severe enough to require disease-modifying antirheumatic drugs (DMARDs). There is no cure for RA, but these drugs can slow the progression of the disease and save the joints and other tissues from permanent damage.

Rheumatic diseases include autoimmune conditions. An autoimmune disease is a condition arising from an abnormal immune response to a normal body part. Any body part can be involved. Essentially the body attacks itself because it mistakenly identifies a body part as a foreign invader like a virus or harmful germ.

There are at least 80 types of autoimmune diseases affecting some 50 million people in the U.S.

They can be broadly divided into two types: those that damage many organs (systemic), and those where only a single organ or tissue is directly damaged by the autoimmune process (localized). In either case, the cause is generally unknown. Some autoimmune diseases tend to run in families and there have been certain cases known to be triggered by infections or other environmental factors. Medical science though, has not found the root cause of most autoimmune disorders.

When the body attacks itself, it causes inflammation. The most common symptoms include low-grade fever and fatigue, which may come and go. With such ambiguous symptoms, it is understandable that diagnosis can be difficult to determine. The most common autoimmune diseases are celiac disease, multiple sclerosis, lupus, inflammatory bowel disease, Graves' disease, psoriasis, fibromyalgia, scleroderma, polymyositis, and vasculitis.

Most rheumatic diseases are inflammatory, but rheumatologists also deal with non-inflammatory conditions like degenerative joint disease, soft tissue and sports related disorders, chronic pain syndromes, and metabolic diseases of the bone. Examples include rickets, achondroplasia, tendinitis, and Marfan's syndrome. There are also many musculoskeletal complications associated with non-rheumatological conditions, such as diabetes mellitus, that are managed by rheumatologists.

Rheumatologists often act in a consulting role to a primary care physician. This usually happens when the patient's condition is limited to a single disorder. It is common, however, for rheumatic conditions to affect multiple systems and organs in the body. In that case, the patient would require an interdisciplinary team of doctors representing different areas of expertise. The rheumatologist would directly manage that healthcare team to ensure that all aspects of the disease are being properly addressed. The rheumatologist would be in charge of the medical records, be the focal point for communications between providers, and make referrals to specialists as needed.

The work of a rheumatologist can be divided into two main parts: diagnosis and treatment. An initial visit to a rheumatologist may include joint examination, blood tests, x-rays, and a general health assessment. When the cause of illness is not readily apparent, other imaging methods may be used, such as an MRI, CT scan, or ultrasound. Some cases need to be confirmed through biopsies.

Once a diagnosis has been determined, the rheumatologist develops and coordinates an individualized treatment plan that may include elements of physiotherapy, occupational therapy, and medications. Drug therapy options include analgesics, steroids, nonsteroidal anti-inflammatory drugs, specialty medications designed for specific disorders, DMARDs, and low-dose chemotherapy. Drugs may be administered orally, by injections, or through infusions.

Rheumatic diseases tend to be chronic, meaning they cannot be cured. They can only be managed. An important part of the rheumatologist's job is educating patients and their families on what to expect and how to cope with a long-term health problem.

Subspecialties

Rheumatology is a specialty of either internal medicine or pediatrics. Internists treat adults, while pediatricians only treat children. Rheumatic and autoimmune diseases affect so many people in so many ways, that there are many rheumatologists who develop interests in highly focused areas such as metabolic bone disease, neurophysiology, or sports medicine. Some specialize in treating a particular type of disease, and some even limit their practice to certain types of patients with a particular type of disease, such as teenagers with Lupus.

Research

Many rheumatologists get involved in research to advance better understanding of the various types of rheumatic disorders, or to help develop better methods of diagnosis or treatment.   A PhD is usually required to qualify for a research position. Many rheumatologist trainees earn a PhD by undertaking two to three years of formal research conducted at their schools.

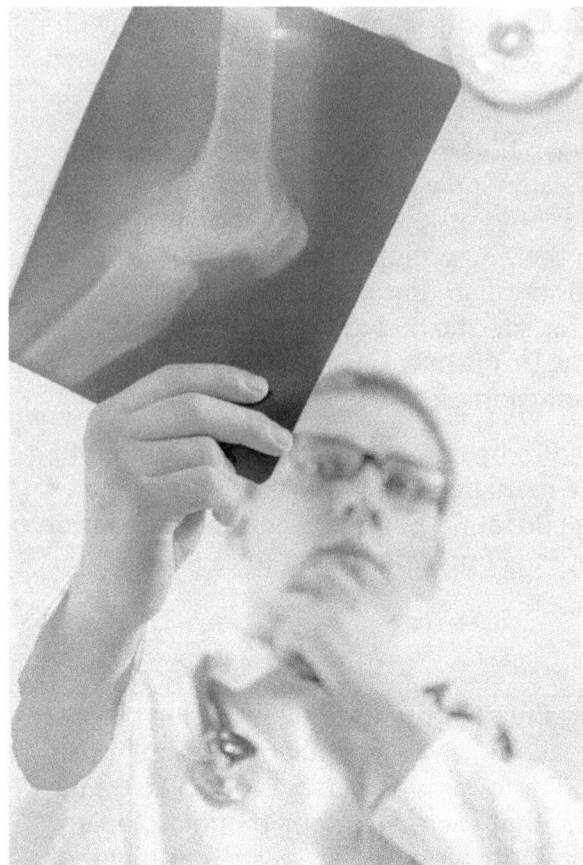

There are many opportunities for rheumatologists to become involved in research. Positions exist in both the public and private sectors. The majority of clinical research, including important clinical trials, is performed at major universities and teaching hospitals. Academic researchers are faculty members and are required to teach classes. Some of the leaders in rheumatology studies include University of California San Francisco, Cedar-Sinai Hospital, UCLA, Cleveland Clinic, Mayo Clinic, U Mass, and the University of Washington. Pure research is conducted by government agencies, such as the National Institutes of Health (NIH). Most research done in the private sector is conducted by pharmaceutical firms in search of new treatments.

STORIES OF WORKING RHEUMATOLOGISTS

I Work with Veterans

"When I first started working at Walter Reed Hospital, I had no idea I wanted to be a rheumatologist. Frankly, I wasn't even sure what rheumatology was. But there was a huge population of patients with inflammatory arthritis and no one with sufficient expertise to treat them. My commanding officer told me to switch my specialty to rheumatology and I did. Now I provide non-surgical care for veterans who have autoimmune and musculoskeletal disorders, such as osteoarthritis, tendinitis, bursitis, gout, fibromyalgia, and vasculitis. My goal is to help improve their quality of life through increased physical function and decreased pain.

It is surprising to me how much enjoyment there is in caring for people who suffer from chronic illness. There is a great deal of satisfaction in helping people control serious health problems over a long period of time. I think the best part of my career in rheumatology has been the development of genuine long-term friendships with patients.

Diagnostic and treatment methods have continually changed over the years. I envision more advances in the future, like medications that can be tailored to each person, based on that individual's unique genetic make-up.

I would suggest that medical students consider a career in the military. There are tremendous opportunities available. VA hospitals in every state are in great need of rheumatologists. I am grateful to my commanding officer for launching my career. I have been very fortunate to have been of service to so many people."

I Am a Pediatric Resident

"During my second year of residency, I had to choose a two-week elective. I chose pediatric rheumatology because I thought it would be simple. I soon realized, however, that my impression of this specialty was completely distorted. Rheumatology may be the only medical specialty where there are more questions than answers. I found myself enjoying the challenge of diagnostic dilemmas and trying to understand the pathophysiology of rheumatic conditions, particularly autoimmune and inflammatory diseases.

I was also fascinated by the effect of these diseases on patients, especially young ones. Children who are hospitalized are naturally scared and how they react is unpredictable. I always keep in mind that they are pleasant kids who just need someone to explain difficult concepts in language they can understand. They also need constant reassurance, much more so than their adult counterparts.

There are many therapies that I can use to make these children and teenagers feel better and function better, and there are more therapies coming along all the time. I am amazed how many breakthroughs have led to better lives for my patients, and the future continues to be bright. I look forward to bringing the advances to my young patients."

I Am an Assistant Professor

"Until my third year of medical school, my plan was to become a surgeon. A rotation in rheumatology changed my mind. I was especially intrigued by immunology and the rapidly advancing science in the field. It seemed new discoveries were being made all the time. They often led to some of the most important cutting-edge advancements in medicine. For example, pharmaceutical companies have developed biological agents that target very specific parts of the immune system. These agents are replacing old treatments, such as chemotherapy drugs, which are less effective and very hard on the body.

Today, I work at a medical school, but my professional identity is that of a clinical rheumatologist. My days are a blend of administrative tasks, teaching, and patient care. No matter what I'm doing, there is great personal and professional satisfaction that I doubt I would have experienced in a surgical career. When I work with patients, I have the chance to make a difference in their lives. When I am teaching, I am providing the world with better, much-needed doctors.

Rheumatology has always provided me with great intellectual stimulation. Exciting scientific advances are continuing to come at a breathtaking pace. The therapeutic options I have available to me now could only be imagined when I entered the field. The diverse nature of rheumatic diseases keeps me sharp as an internist.

The relationships I have with my patients are special. They are long term, and therefore require a solid foundation of mutual respect one does not see in other clinical specialties. I consider it a privilege to be able to make such a tremendous positive impact in the lives of so many people devastated by disabling, deforming diseases. It is undoubtedly the most appealing aspect of my work.

Anyone considering this career should know that there is a nationwide shortage of trained rheumatologists due to an increasing incidence of musculoskeletal and autoimmune diseases in our country. At the same time, there is improved reimbursement for practicing rheumatologists. This specialty offers a great opportunity to practice anywhere and enjoy a comfortable lifestyle."

PERSONAL QUALITIES

RHEUMATOLOGY CAN BE AN EXCELLENT CHOICE for individuals who are very interested in a career in medicine. It is a fast-paced job that requires great organizational skills, a passion for problem solving, and a strong desire to help people who are struggling to maintain normal lives. Employers hiring rheumatologists typically look for certain qualities in job candidates.

Compassion

Rheumatologists must have excellent bedside manners and the ability to help patients feel at ease. Rheumatology patients often suffer from painful and debilitating conditions. They need to be treated with warmth and respect. Most rheumatic illnesses are lifelong conditions, which means you will be developing relationships with patients and their families that will last for years. Every day, you will be working with all kinds of people from every age group and background. It takes a real people person with outstanding interpersonal skills to earn their trust.

Communications Skills

Excellent communications skills are critical in this field. You should be comfortable talking to all kinds of people, including children, adults from all education levels, and other healthcare professionals. It is especially important to be able to provide information in layman terms that patients and their families can understand. Listening is just as important as talking. Excellent listening skills will allow you to better relate to people and assess their situations more quickly.

Easygoing Nature

This work can be stressful, but you must remain calm. People with rheumatic ailments often suffer painful conditions that are unrelenting. They naturally can be very irritable and frustrated, especially when their treatments do not appear to be working. The problem is even worse with children, particularly those who are too young for deep discussions. It helps to have a positive attitude and a great deal of patience.

Cooperation

Rheumatologists should be able to get along well with others and work effectively as part of a team. Although much of their time is spent working one-on-one with patients, rheumatologists are often consulted by other healthcare providers. A spirit of cooperation will go a long way towards providing complete coordinated care for patients.

Determination

There are more than 200 kinds of rheumatic diseases and more are being discovered all the time. Many share similar symptoms that make them hard to differentiate. Others are so rare, they are difficult to diagnose. It can sometimes take months to correctly identify the condition and even more time to get a handle on the best treatment plan. Successful rheumatologists are always prepared to go the distance for their patients. You will need to stay focused while continually providing reassurance to patients who may be frustrated and scared.

Intellectual Curiosity

This is especially important for those going into research, but all rheumatologists must be willing to keep up with information that is continually evolving. There are new diseases being identified, improved diagnostic techniques, and hundreds of clinical drug trials underway at any given moment. Medical school lays a good foundation, but it is only the start. The best rheumatologists are avid readers, eager to learn new things that will help them treat their patients more effectively.

ATTRACTIVE FEATURES

IF YOU ARE LOOKING FOR A SECURE FUTURE in a career that will make you happy, you have come to the right place. You will need to invest a considerable amount of time, money, and hard work to get the necessary training, but there will be a payoff upon graduation. There are more than enough jobs for all qualified candidates, the pay is great, and there is little chance of career burnout. Rheumatologists also enjoy a balanced life, the satisfaction of changing work patters, and building long-term relationships with their patients. For these reasons, Medicare found that rheumatologists are the happiest specialists after polling more than 292,000 doctors of all kinds.

Rheumatologists make good money. In fact, they make five times the median income of US households, and roughly $40,000 a year more than the average for all physicians. There are specialists who earn more, but they tend to be the ones who are less happy in their careers. Even new rheumatologists are paid well. Entry-level incomes range from $120,000 to around $180,000, and with some years of experience that can rise to nearly $300,000. Pay is going up steadily as demand for services grows faster than the supply of qualified rheumatologists.

The job outlook is excellent. Opportunities are plentiful, even at the entry level, and the future looks even brighter. The incidence of rheumatic diseases is growing much faster than the number of rheumatologists entering the field. A mere 2.8 percent of internal medicine residents are electing to go into rheumatology. That is expected to create a shortage of 2,600 rheumatologists by 2025. That amounts to a 50 percent increase in the shortfall!

Rheumatologists get to form long-term relationships with their patients. Rheumatic diseases are chronic, meaning they are never cured. They have to be managed for a lifetime. Patients often become a big part of a rheumatologist's life through the years. Only family doctors enjoy the same kind of relationships that rheumatologists form with patients and their families.

Rheumatologists find a great deal of personal and professional satisfaction in their work. Patients come in the door experiencing various levels of pain. Some are in pain so extreme they can hardly get out of bed. Others are not able to carry out the usual functions of daily life. The treatments that are available today can ease pain and make it possible for a person to return to a normal life. Who would not be happy about changing lives in such a positive way?

Smart people love this work, especially those who like solving puzzles. Rheumatology is the specialty that other doctors turn to when no one else can figure out what is going on. Rheumatic diseases can be difficult to diagnose. Symptoms can be vague and enigmatic. They often mimic numerous other diseases. Rheumatologists take pride in diagnosing complex conditions, some of which are not even rheumatic. The work is often challenging, but it is always intellectually stimulating, whether you are researching possible cures in a laboratory or working with patients in clinical settings.

UNATTRACTIVE ASPECTS

RHEUMATOLOGY CAN BE A VERY FULFILLING CAREER with a salary well into six figures, but like any career, there are pros and cons to be considered. The most obvious downside of rheumatology is the lengthy education requirements. Even if you start your training immediately after high school, you will be well into your 30s before you start practicing. All those years of schooling come at a cost, too. Many years of education result in massive student loans to pay back. On the plus side, even a new rheumatologist earns enough right away to start loan repayment without having to resort to a diet based on ramen noodles.

The hours can be long. It is not unusual for rheumatologists to work more than 60 hours a week. Rheumatologists who work in hospitals may need to work weekends or be on call. That kind of schedule can wreak havoc with your social life. Some find it hard to establish a family. Others only socialize with the people they see at work.

The work can be tiring. Rheumatologists are on their feet most of the day. Working more than 60 hours can be exhausting. Still, no matter how tired you are, you have to stay focused to avoid mistakes that could negatively affect a patient's life.

Career advancement is almost nonexistent in rheumatology. There is no career ladder to climb. Once you are a practicing rheumatologist, that is your position. A few might become department heads, but most will need to be happy with a position that will always stay essentially the same.

There is a mountain of paperwork, especially for those in private practice. There are pre-authorization forms for medications and diagnostic studies, as well as a huge pile of documentation associated with electronic health records. Keeping up with all the bureaucratic tasks can be stressful. Not only is it tedious, it takes time away from seeing patients.

Some medical specialties are cooler than others. Rheumatology cannot really compete with the image of a surgeon performing open-heart surgery, removing a brain tumor, or sewing a hand back on, all while casually chatting to the nurses and residents around the operating table. Maybe that is why rheumatology attracts so few new recruits. Rheumatology seems rather low key and lacking in drama, but these doctors do earn the undying respect and gratitude of millions of patients who lead better lives thanks to their work.

EDUCATION AND TRAINING

A DOCTORAL DEGREE IS THE EDUCATIONAL REQUIREMENT for entry-level rheumatologists. To become a practicing rheumatologist, an undergraduate degree (four years), medical school (four years), residency training (three years), and fellowship training (two years) are required. That is a minimum of 13 years of intense education before one can be licensed to practice. There is no shortcut.

It is normal for students to start out either not knowing what kind of medicine they would want to practice, or they think they know, but change their mind after being introduced to other possibilities. Most are not even exposed to rheumatology until the second or third year of medical school. According to a survey by the American College of Rheumatology, more than 75 percent of medical students make the decision to specialize in rheumatology during their residency program – which comes after graduating from medical school.

Rheumatologists can be either medical doctors (MDs) or osteopathic doctors (DOs). A doctor's credentials will indicate which. A medical doctor will be a Fellow of the American College of Rheumatology (FACR). An osteopathic rheumatologist will be a Fellow of the American Osteopathic College of Rheumatology (FAOCR). Both are qualified to practice rheumatology and are licensed by the same state licensing boards. They both follow the same academic path, though they attend different schools. DOs receive their medical degrees from osteopathic schools, while MDs graduate from medical schools. DOs do have to take 200 more hours of training to learn manipulation techniques of the musculoskeletal system. Other than that, there is little, if any, difference in their education.

Undergraduate Studies

A medical education starts with an undergraduate degree, which is usually a bachelor's degree that takes four years to complete. Many undergraduate students pursue a pre-med program, which places heavy emphasis on the sciences, such as physics, biology, and chemistry, both inorganic and organic. However, pre-med is not the only choice. Other majors may qualify for admission to medical school as long as they include classes related to human anatomy, general sciences, medicine, or biology.

In the junior or senior year, undergraduate students can take the Medical College Admissions Test (MCAT). Administered by the AAMC (Association of American Medical Colleges), it is a standardized, multiple-choice exam created to help medical schools determine if you have the requisite critical thinking skills, knowledge of scientific concepts, and aptitude to study medicine. Almost all medical schools in the US and Canada require applicants to submit MCAT exam scores. Admissions officers also look for letters of recommendation, good grades, and an essay. Doing some volunteer work in the medical field is also helpful.

Medical School

Once you have been admitted to medical school, you can expect four years of intensive instruction and clinical rotations. During the first two years (M1 and M2), classroom instruction covers subjects such as anatomy, biochemistry, physiology, microbiology, pharmacology, psychology, and medical ethics. The remaining two years (M3 and M4) provide instruction and training through rotations in different specialties.

Rotations, which typically last four to eight weeks, take place at hospitals and clinics affiliated with the school. They are designed to provide exposure to various medical specialties, such as pediatrics, surgery, psychiatry, and internal medicine etc. The goal is to help students decide which area of medicine to focus on. Students learn how to care for patients within real medical settings while under the supervision of experienced doctors. They learn how to check patients, diagnose medical conditions, and take a medical history.

Residency

After graduating from medical school, students will need to complete a three-year residency program (it is longer in some other specialties). At this point, it is necessary to decide between treating adults or treating children. If you want to treat children, you would choose a residency in pediatrics. For treating adults, the residency would be internal medicine. Residency programs, which consist of hands-on training, are conducted primarily in hospital settings.

Residents work long hours. Twelve to 16 hour days are normal, and they can go even longer when on call. The time is spent diagnosing symptoms, reviewing lab tests, scrutinizing patient vital signs, and developing and evaluating treatment plans.

Licensing

In the US, all doctors are required to obtain a license in order to practice. After you have completed the first year of residency (which was formerly call an internship), you can apply for a license in the state where you intend to practice. You are then legally a doctor, although most physicians continue and complete their residency.

Fellowship

After finishing a residency program, rheumatologists spend an additional two or three years in a fellowship program. Fellowship programs are affiliated with universities. They provide extensive exposure to current theory and clinical practice. Participants learn from faculty experts in areas such as immunology, applied basic laboratory research, clinical rheumatology, and the epidemiology and outcomes of rheumatic diseases. The purpose of fellowship programs is to hone the skills of new rheumatologists and prepare them for careers in research or clinical practice.

Certification

Most rheumatologists become board certified. Board certification makes a rheumatologist more employable and assures patients that the doctor has the knowledge and ongoing training necessary to provide a high level of care. To become certified in rheumatology, applicants must:

- Already be certified in internal medicine or pediatrics

- Complete the requisite two or three years of fellowship training

- Demonstrate clinical competence, procedural skills, and ethical behavior

- Hold a valid license to practice medicine

- Pass a rheumatology certification exam

Rheumatologists treating adults take the exam administered by the American Board of Internal Medicine, while rheumatologists treating children take the exam given by the American Board of Pediatrics.

A recertification process is required every 10 years. During that time, it is necessary to attend continuing education courses and conferences. It is through this ongoing training that rheumatologists stay on top of advances in the practice of rheumatology, and learn about new approaches and treatments for various patient conditions.

EARNINGS

RHEUMATOLOGISTS ARE PAID WELL. The lowest salaries are paid to new professionals. Entry-level earnings average about $180,000, but that is just a starting point. Every year in practice, a rheumatologist's salary grows. With some years of experience, the annual salary can be as high as $350,000. Earnings are expected to go even higher in the future.

In addition to experience, salaries for rheumatologists vary most by geographical location and self-employment versus salaried staff.

According to the most recent survey by Medicare, the highest annual salaries for rheumatologists are currently found in the Southeast and South Central regions. The lowest are in the Northwest and Mid-Atlantic. Regardless of location, however, competition and physician density play a role in rheumatologists' salaries.

As a general rule, rheumatologists make more money in private practice than those who work on staff in other work environments, such as hospitals, healthcare organizations, and government agencies. The difference in earnings is roughly $40,000 a year, but anyone considering self-employment has to take into account the cost of being self-employed. Overhead includes rent and utilities, payroll, insurance, license and operation fees, furniture, and equipment (both office and medical). Start-up costs also need to include living expenses for the first few months while building a patient base.

There are also differences among various work settings. For example, the average income for rheumatologists in a multi-specialty group practice is about $235,000, while it is about $185,000 for those on staff in hospitals. All the top earners are in private practice. Those who earn the least money are employed by healthcare organizations and academic and government centers.

In addition to generous salaries, most employers offer a great benefits package. Some of the benefits include:

- Paid vacation and sick days
- Paid holidays or double time pay for those who choose to work
- Pension and/or 401k plans
- Profit sharing
- Bonuses paid quarterly or annually
- Long and short term disability insurance
- Life and medical insurance that can include family members
- Vision and dental coverage

Other perks may include reimbursement for continuing education, paid malpractice insurance, cell phone for those on call, and paid travel expenses when going to seminars and conferences.

Those who are self-employed must provide their own benefits, not only to themselves, but also to any employees in their practice.

OPPORTUNITIES

THE CURRENT JOB MARKET IS VERY GOOD for rheumatologists and the outlook for the future looks promising as well. Job growth for all types of doctors is expected to grow 14 percent over the coming decade. Rheumatologists can anticipate even greater job growth, partly because there is a relatively small percentage of doctors who specialize in this field of medicine. Those with extensive experience will enjoy the best prospects, but even beginners will find plenty of opportunities.

Many job openings will result from attrition. Most rheumatologists today are between 50 and 60 years old. That means a significant portion of the workforce will be retiring over the next 15 years. Others will be transferring to other specialties or leaving the field for a variety of personal reasons, such as illness or death. There are not enough trainees preparing to enter the field to fill all the vacancies.

The growing and aging population is expected to drive overall job growth. The US population is continually growing and it is getting older, too, because people (on average) are living longer. Rheumatic ailments, such as arthritis, are common among older adults. The Baby Boom generation, in particular, is experiencing an increase of musculoskeletal diseases, including rheumatoid arthritis and osteoarthritis. The prevalence of disease will create a strong demand for specialists who treat rheumatic conditions.

There are not enough rheumatologists to keep up with the need. There are more than 100 diseases specifically classified as rheumatic, including many types of arthritis. According to the Centers for Disease Control and Prevention (CDC), these diseases afflict more than 53 million Americans. Rheumatologists are also responsible for diagnosing and treating autoimmune diseases, which account for the fastest growing area of illness in the US. Currently, there are 50 million Americans suffering from autoimmune diseases. That is roughly 20 percent of the population, or one in five people who are diagnosed with diseases like lupus, celiac disease, vasculitis, fibromyalgia, Crohn's, and type 1 diabetes.

As of now, there are approximately 5200 rheumatologists in the US. That is not nearly enough to care for the number of people in need of these services. According to a study conducted by the American College of Rheumatology, there is an anticipated increase in demand for rheumatology services of 45 percent through the year 2025. At the same time, the number of new graduates entering the workforce is expected to remain constant. The result is a significant gap between supply and demand. According to a study by Johns Hopkins, there needs to be 7,210 adult rheumatologists by 2025, which represents a shortfall of 2,576. The shortfall is less for pediatric rheumatologists, but it is still significant. In short, there are many people who will need the specific services that only rheumatologists can provide, who will be underserved.

There are jobs everywhere, but as with most medical specialties, the need is greater in less populated areas. Those who want to work in major metropolitan areas might run into some competition for the best jobs. Those looking in small to medium sized cities and rural areas will have very little difficulty finding employment or opportunities for private practice.

GETTING STARTED

START LAYING THE GROUNDWORK FOR YOUR CAREER long before you graduate. First, you should investigate your options to determine what career path to take. Do you want to go into private practice or be on staff at a hospital? Are you interested in research? Or maybe teaching is your passion. Whatever area you choose to focus on will guide your activities as you prepare to step into the real world of medicine.

It is important to get as much hands-on experience as possible while still in school. Internships are an integral component of every medical school program. Try to participate in as many internships as you can. Look for volunteer opportunities, too. Community health centers, assisted living facilities, and hospitals always need extra help. In addition to gaining valuable experience, take advantage of these opportunities to start networking. Always strive to do more than what is expected of you and offer to take on extra responsibilities. You will make a lasting impression that will pay off in the years to come.

Networking is key to a successful career. Start gathering contacts and references right away. Your first networking contacts will be your professors, but there are many other sources. Attend seminars at your school, outside industry conferences, workshops, and meetings. Each of these activities provides excellent opportunities to interact with established professionals who can help you get started on your career path. Take advantage of the question and answer sessions that usually follow these kinds of events to get answers to your most pressing questions while making yourself known to prospective contacts.

Join professional associations. Most rheumatologists belong to more than one. In addition to providing job leads, these organizations represent a great source of networking possibilities. There are more than 9,000 rheumatology health professionals who belong to the American College of Rheumatology (ACR) alone. Be sure to check out all the membership benefits, such as educational discounts, research opportunities, fellowships, and access to the latest information on rheumatology-related topics. Be an active member. Attend meetings, join committees, and interact socially. Rheumatology is a small universe. Through active participation, you will eventually meet just about everyone in your field.

Aside from networking, there are several other good ways to find your first position. Your school's career center will have listings of job openings. Check with your professors, too, especially the department head. Hospitals and research centers often have relationships with faculty members. Opportunities are often filled by tapping referrals. In fact, many are never advertised or listed on a job board.

Contact employment agencies, both on the Internet and off. There are many that specialize in healthcare jobs. You can also apply directly to potential employers such as hospitals, clinics, laboratories, and private medical practices. Keep your résumé polished and ready, complete with letters of recommendation from professors and supervisors. Subscribe to medical journals and other publications that cater to the field of rheumatology. Be a well-informed job candidate by staying abreast on the current issues and trends related to the management and treatment of rheumatic diseases.

ASSOCIATIONS

■ **American College of Rheumatology**
http://www.rheumatology.org

■ **The Association of American Medical Colleges (AAMC)**
https://www.aamc.org

■ **The American Society of Clinical Rheumatologists**
http://www.ascr.us

■ **The National Organization of Rheumatology Managers**
https://www.normgroup.org

■ **Arthritis Foundation**
http://www.arthritis.org

■ **Rheumatology Research Foundation**
www.rheumresearch.org

PERIODICAL

■ **The Rheumatologist**
http://www.the-rheumatologist.org